# GET
## THAT
# WORK

MARCUS WEBB

NEWMAN SPRINGS PUBLISHING
320 Broad Street
Red Bank, NJ 07701

First originally published by Newman Springs Publishing 2023

ISBN 979-8-88763-640-5 (Paperback)
ISBN 979-8-88763-641-2 (Digital)

Printed in the United States of America

My name is Marcus Webb. I'm a certified fitness trainer and boxing coach. I have been in the fitness industry for over thirty years. I have coached a wide variety of individuals from housewives, kids, general workers, police officers, doctors, attorneys, military staff to premium athletes. I can create an effective fitness program for anyone. I have a fitness certification from *International Fitness Association* and a boxing coach certification from the legendary Tony Spain, a former Golden Glove champion.

The reason for this e-book is to coach, instruct, and teach individuals how to perform various exercises. The e-book also provides you with information on eating plans/diets, supplemental information, workout programs, kickboxing drills, motivation quotes, and testimonials from fitness clients I have coached and am still coaching.

A portion of the book proceeds will go to help me continue to offer free fitness training to young athletes going to college and continue to purchase essential kits for the homeless.

# Estimated food calorie list

One chicken breast—165 calories
One salmon—180 calories
One steak—300 calories
One cup ground turkey—240 calories
Grilled chicken salad with dressing—650 calories
One strip of turkey bacon—30 calories
One cup of cooked oatmeal—160 calories
One boiled or scrambled egg—85 calories
One piece of toast—75 calories
One sweet potato—115 calories
One cup broccoli—30 calories
One spear of asparagus—3 calories
One cup of cooked rice—205 calories
One avocado—250 calories
One protein shake—100 calories

# Eating plans/diets

Breakfast—protein shake
Lunch—protein shake
Snack—fruits or nuts
Dinner—a protein, a veggie, and a carb
Snack—protein shake or fruit/nuts

# Intermittent fasting low-carb eating plan

11:00 a.m.—oatmeal, four egg whites, four strips of turkey bacon
1:00 p.m.—avocado, almonds, blueberries, or protein shake
3:00 p.m.—chicken breast or baked fish or turkey tenderloin with sweet potato and broccoli
5:00 p.m.—avocado, almonds, blueberries, or protein shake
7:00 p.m.—chicken breast or baked fish or turkey tenderloin with sweet potato and broccoli

# Three-thousand-calorie eating plan

Meal 1—three whole eggs with either 1 cup of grits or 1 cup oatmeal
Meal 2—either protein shake with 1 scoop carbs or 6 oz chicken breast and 1/2 cup rice
Meal 3—either 6 oz of chicken breast or ground chicken/turkey with 1/2 cup rice and veggies
Meal 4—protein shake and either one apple or one banana
Meal 5—either 6 oz of fish, beef, or chicken with either 1/2 cup rice or one sweet potato with veggies

# Foods that help curb hunger

Eggs, coffee, strawberries, pickles, carrots, seltzer, broccoli, cottage cheese, salads, green tea, watermelon, Greek yogurt, tuna, soup, protein powder, oats.

# Calories in alcohol

Beer—125 calories
Champagne—96 calories
Wine—125 calories
Whiskey—105 calories
Vodka—96 calories
Gin and tonic—190 calories
Tequila—69 calories

# Weight-gain eating plan

Breakfast—700 calories
1 cup oatmeal
3 boiled or scrambled eggs
2 strips of turkey bacon
2 slices of toast
1 avocado
Protein shake

Lunch—650 calories
Grilled chicken salad with dressing
or
2 chicken breasts
1 sweet potato
3 cups broccoli
Protein shake

Dinner—650–800 calories
2 chicken breasts
1 sweet potato
1 cup broccoli
5 spears asparagus
1 avocado
or
Steak
1 sweet potato
1 cup broccoli
1 avocado
or
1 cup ground turkey
1 sweet potato
1 cup broccoli
1 avocado

or
2 pieces of salmon
1 sweet potato
1 cup broccoli
5 spears of asparagus
1 avocado

## Morning fuel

Eggs, coffee, Greek yogurt, protein shake, oatmeal, fruits/berries, flax/chia seeds, cottage cheese.

## Muscle recovery 101

Carbs and protein powder, get sleep, yoga, foam rolling, stay hydrated, warm bath, massage, and walking.

## Great sources of protein

Chicken breast, ground turkey, ground beef, steak, tofu, lentils, quinoa, beans, Greek yogurt, cottage cheese, egg whites, whey protein, tuna, salmon, shrimp, and cod.

## Foods for stomachache

White rice, ginger, white toast, coconut water, banana, oats, papaya, apple, and potatoes.

## Foods that contain almost zero calories

Garlic, broccoli, carrots, cucumber, tomatoes, spinach, watermelon, apples, cauliflower, and celery.

# Know your macros

Carbs—rice, oats, bread, pasta, cereal, veggie, potatoes, whole grains, whole wheat.

Proteins—fish, whey, tofu, pork, turkey, chicken, beef, Greek yogurt, egg whites.

Fats—nuts, olives, cheese, olive oil, avocado, egg yolk, flaxseeds, chia seeds.

# Energy-boosting foods

Beets, broccoli, green tea, eggs, dark chocolate, almonds, sweet potatoes, dandelion leaf, and raspberry leaf.

# Cancer-fighting foods

Green tea, blackberries, raspberries, blueberries, lemons, onions, kale, green leafy veggies, turmeric, artichokes, garlic, tomatoes, olive oil, dark chocolate, oregano, ginger, cauliflower, Brussel sprouts, avocado, nuts/seeds, broccoli, mushrooms, ginseng, carrots, jalapeños, figs, flax, great fruit, red grapes, red wine, rosemary, and seaweed.

## Cardio fat-loss and endurance workout

Do eight one-minute sprints.
One minute: 7.5 mph
One minute: 7.7 mph
One minute: 8.0 mph
One minute: 8.3 mph
One minute: 8.5 mph
One minute: 8.7 mph
One minute: 8.8 mph
One minute: 9.0 mph

## Total body barbell workout

Sixty push-ups
Sixty hanging knee raises
Sixty chest presses
Sixty RDLs
Sixty standing shoulder presses
Eight-one minute sprints
Sixty push-ups
Sixty hanging knee raises
Sixty bicep barbell curls
Sixty barbell squats
Sixty close-grip triceps presses

## Bodyweight workout

Ten push-ups
Twenty squats
Ten burpees
Twenty lunges
One-minute mountain climbers
One-minute planks
Perform four sets

## Bodyweight workout

Do each exercise for thirty seconds/rest for thirty seconds in between each exercise.

Perform two to three sets.

Jumping jacks
Air jumps
Mountain climbers
Military squats
Butt kicks
Plank rolls
Standing lunges
Half burpees
Jogging
Push-ups

# Fat-burning workout

Five-minute stair climber
Twenty-five push-ups—two times
Twenty-five reverse ab crunches—two times
Twenty barbell chest bench presses—two times
Twenty barbell dead lifts—two times
Twenty shoulder shrugs—two times
HIIT cardio one-minute sprints—eight times
Twenty-five push-ups—two times
Twenty-five reverse ab crunches—two times
Twenty barbell bicep curls—two times
Twenty tricep dips—two times
Twenty (deep) barbell leg squats—two times

# One hour beast mode fit workout

Three one-minute sprints
Fifty hanging knee raises
Fifty push-ups
Fifty bench chest presses
Fifty shoulder shrugs
Fifty lat pulls
Five one-minute sprints
Fifty hanging knee raises
Fifty push-ups
Fifty tricep dips
Fifty barbell curls
Fifty leg presses/fifty calf presses

# Get ripped with HIIT (perform each exercise for thirty seconds)

Jump lunges
Tricep dips
Jumping jacks
Rest thirty seconds
Push-ups
Jump squats
Russian twist
Rest thirty seconds
Mountain climbers
Speed skaters
Planks

# MMA workout

One thousand punches
Five hundred kicks
One hundred push-ups
One hundred squats
One hundred sit-ups
One hundred pull-ups
One hundred lunges
Fifty burpees
Fifty box jumps
Five-minute planks

# Old-school (running the rack) dumbbell exercise

You can perform this workout for your chest, biceps, shoulders, back, legs, abs, and triceps.

40-lb dumbbells—fifteen reps
45-lb dumbbells—twelve reps
50-lb dumbbells—ten reps
45-lb dumbbells—twelve reps
40-lb dumbbells—fifteen reps
A total of sixty-four reps.

# Spell-your-name workout

A. Fifty jumping jacks
B. Twenty crunches
C. Thirty squats
D. Fifteen push-ups
E. One-minute wall sits
F. Ten burpees
G. Twenty-second arm circles
H. Twenty squats
I. Thirty jumping jacks
J. Fifteen crunches
K. Ten push-ups
L. Two-minute wall sit
M. Twenty burpees
N. Forty jumping jacks
O. Twenty-five burpees
P. Fifteen arm circles
Q. Thirty crunches
R. Fifteen push-ups
S. Thirty burpees
T. Fifteen squats
U. Thirty-second arm circles
V. Three-minute wall sit
W. Twenty burpees
X. Sixty jumping jacks
Y. Ten crunches
Z. Twenty push-ups

# Bodyweight HIIT workout

Fifty jumping jacks
Fifty high knees
Fifty mountain climbers
Twenty squats
Ten burpees
Twenty-five full sit-ups
Thirty-second plank
Rest
Fifty jumping jacks
Twenty lunges
Fifteen push-ups
Twenty squats
Fifteen tricep dips
Twenty-five crunches
Thirty-second plank
Rest
Fifty jumping jacks
Twenty cross-body punches
Twenty donkey kicks (ten each side)
Twenty squats
Twenty-five Russian twists
Twenty-five bicycle crunches
Thirty-second plank

# CrossFit workout

For time-
Thirty burpees
Thirty dead lifts
Thirty burpees
Thirty cleans
Thirty burpees
Thirty push presses
Thirty burpees
Thirty strict presses
Thirty jerks
Thirty burpees
Thirty kettlebell swings
Thirty burpees
Thirty snatches (left hand)
Thirty burpees
Thirty snatches (right hand)

# Beast mode fit thirty-minute workout

Barbell chest presses—twenty-five reps—two times
Barbell Roman dead lifts—twenty-five reps—two times
Barbell shoulder shrugs—twenty-five reps—two times
Barbell bicep curls—twenty-five reps—two times
Tricep dips—twenty-five reps—two times
Leg presses—twenty-five reps—two times
Calf presses—twenty-five reps—two times
Five one-minute sprints

# Motivational quotes

Some days it's not about health or building muscle. It's just therapy.

This month's diet is next month's body.

Be a wolf.
Be a lion.
Set goals.
Smash them.
Be stronger.
Be better.
Show people who you are.
Never apologize for being awesome.
Stay positive.
Stay the course.

# Eight powerful phrases for the day

1. Believe in yourself
2. Stay strong
3. Never give up
4. Be grateful
5. Work hard
6. Stay humble
7. Be kind
8. Keep smiling

If it doesn't challenge you, it doesn't change you.

Thirty percent gym, 70 percent diet. Abs are made in the kitchen, not the gym.

Train like an athlete, eat like a nutritionist, sleep like a baby, win like a champion.

Never underestimate your strength; never overestimate your weakness.

Every accomplishment starts with the decision to try.

Don't be the same, be better.

Crawling is acceptable; falling is acceptable; puking is acceptable; crying is acceptable; bleeding is acceptable; pain is acceptable; *quitting is not*!

The body achieves what the mind believes.

Never quit. You stumble, get back up. What happened yesterday no longer matters. Today's another day, so get back on track and move closer to your dreams and goals. You can do it.

One should eat to live, not live to eat.

Work out. Eat well. Be patient. Your body will reward you.

Believe you can, and you are halfway there.

You are your only limit.

Your mind will quit a thousand times before your body will. Feel the fear and do it anyway.

What you eat in private is what you eventually wear in public. Eat clean. Look lean.

You cannot exercise your way out of a bad diet.

Be strong. You never know who you're inspiring.

# Top ten reasons to be fit

Boost your brain power.
Melt away stress.
Feel younger.
Improve your health.
Have more energy.
Improve your confidence.
Build relationships.
It's the best antidepressant.
Become an inspiration to others.
Become unstoppable.

Invest in yourself first. Expect nothing from no one and be willing to work for everything.

A goal without a plan is just a wish.

Failure isn't falling down; it's remaining where you've fallen.

Doing crunches and continuing to eat poorly is like detailing your car and continuing to drive in the mud.

You can never expect to succeed if you only put in work on the days you feel like it.

Fitness is not about being better than someone else; it's about being better than you use to be.

Until you get your nutrition right, nothing is going to change.

You are only confined by the walls you build yourself.

Your diet is number one! You can live in the gym, but if you don't eat clean, you're wasting your time.

Discipline is doing what needs to be done, even if you don't want to.

One pound of fat is 3,500 calories. If you want to lose one pound per week, then just burn five hundred calories per day, more than you eat. Weight loss is science, not magic.

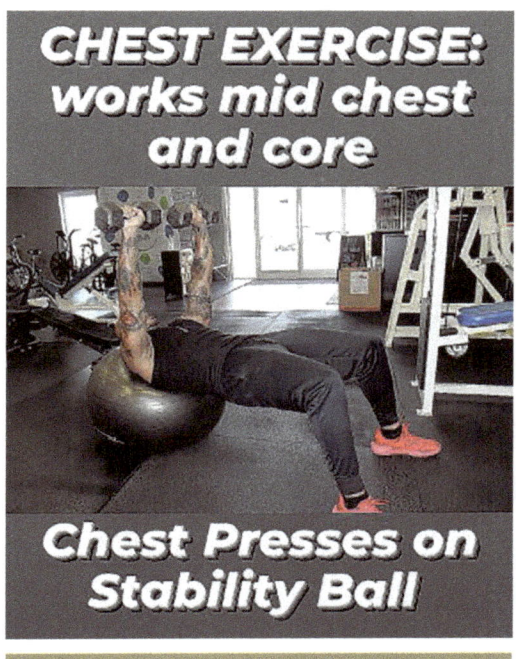

**CHEST EXERCISE: works mid chest and core**

**Chest Presses on Stability Ball**

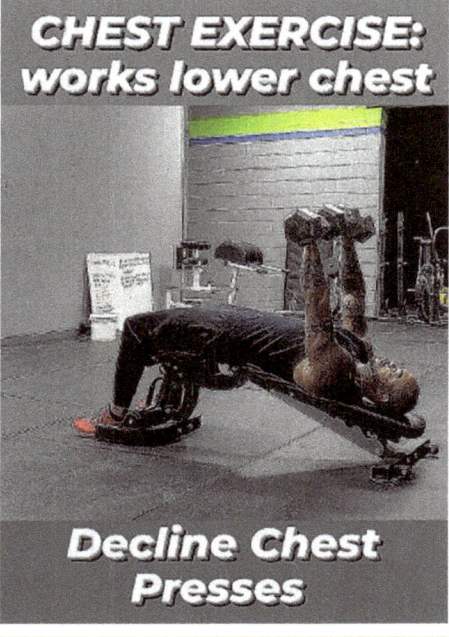

**CHEST EXERCISE: works lower chest**

**Decline Chest Presses**

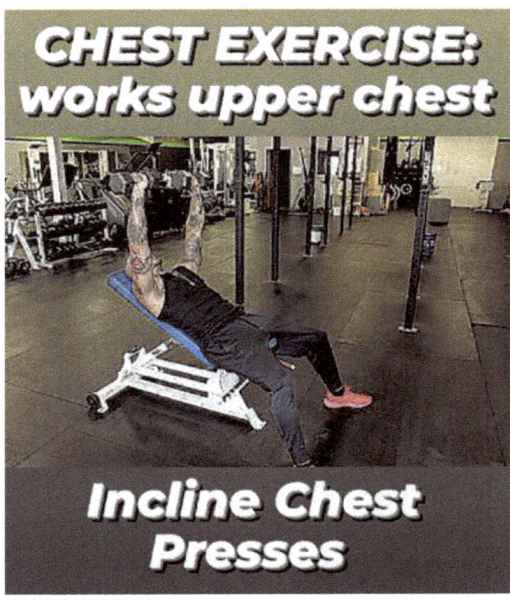

**CHEST EXERCISE: works upper chest**

**Incline Chest Presses**

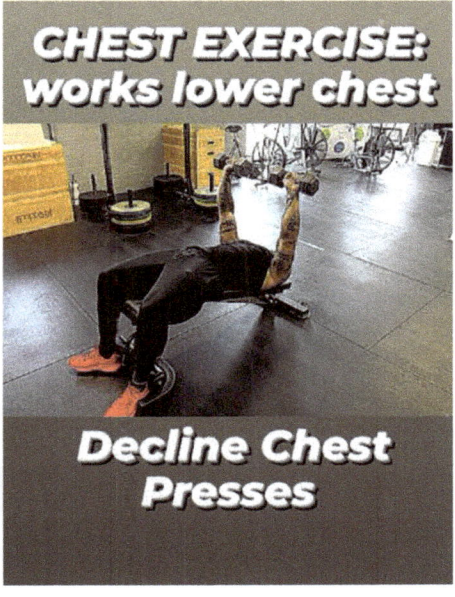

**CHEST EXERCISE: works lower chest**

**Decline Chest Presses**

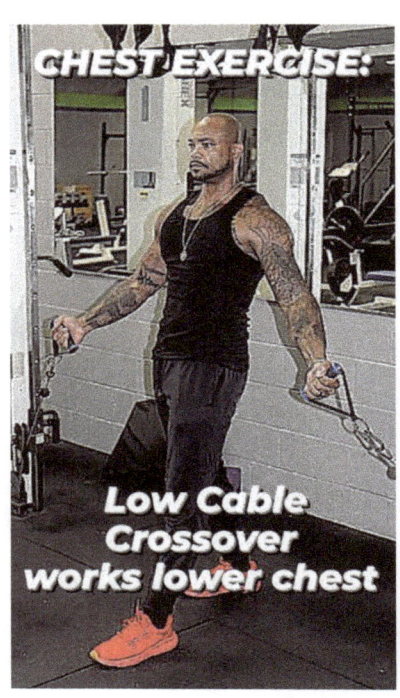

**CHEST EXERCISE:**

Low Cable Crossover works lower chest

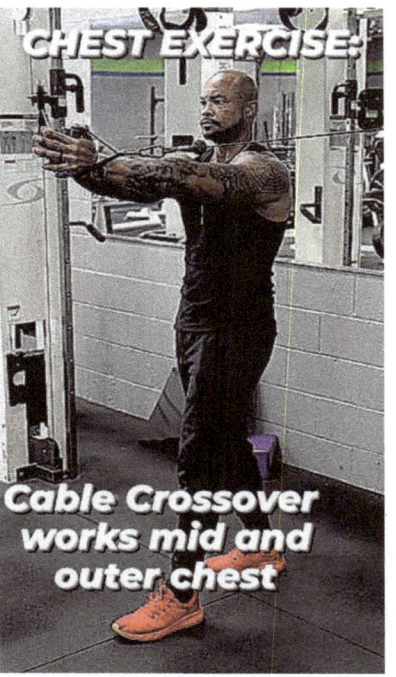

**CHEST EXERCISE:**

Cable Crossover works mid and outer chest

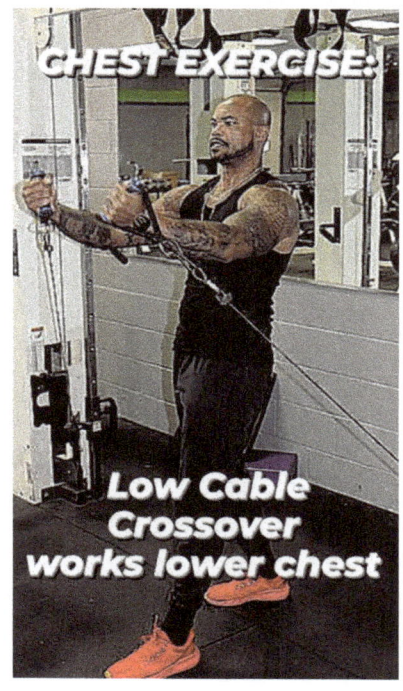

**CHEST EXERCISE:**

Low Cable Crossover works lower chest

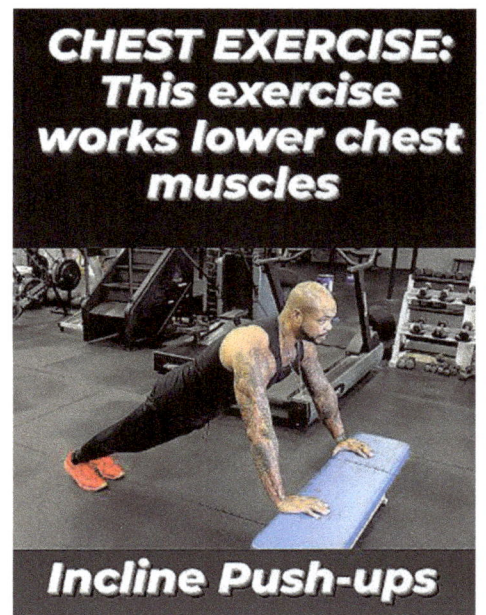

**CHEST EXERCISE:**
This exercise works lower chest muscles

Incline Push-ups

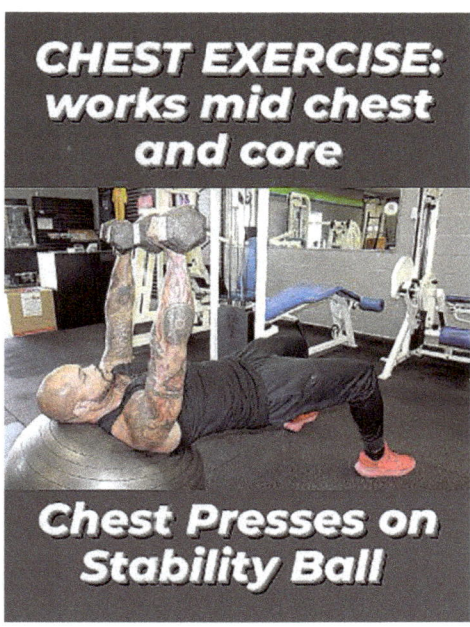

**CHEST EXERCISE:**
works mid chest and core

Chest Presses on Stability Ball

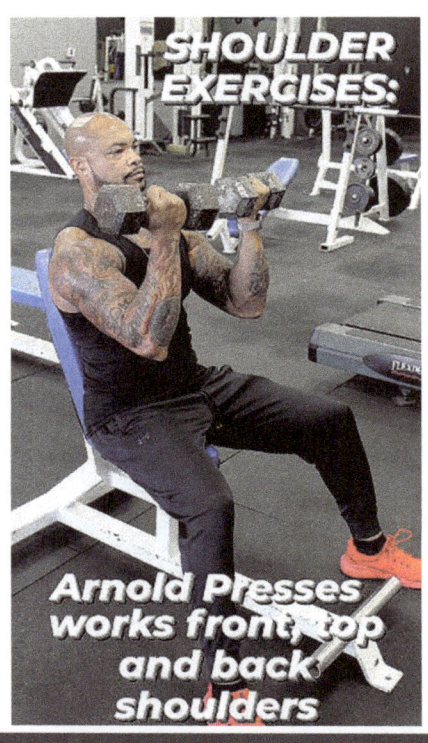

**SHOULDER EXERGISES:**

**Arnold Presses works front, top and back shoulders**

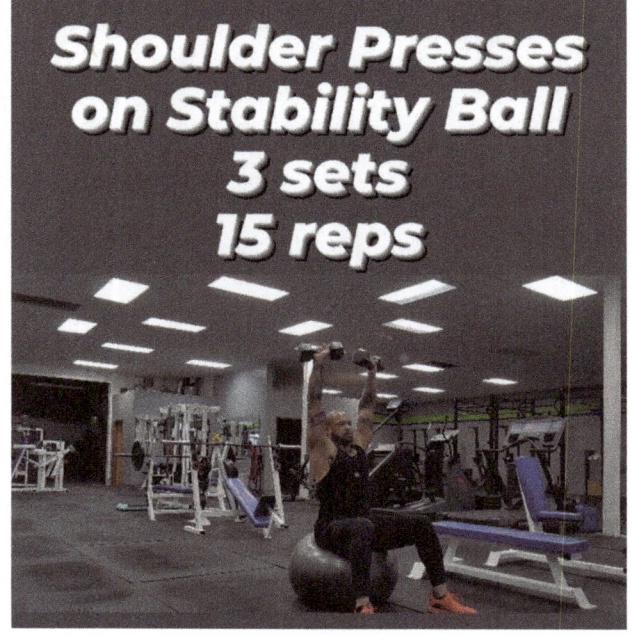

**Shoulder Presses on Stability Ball
3 sets
15 reps**

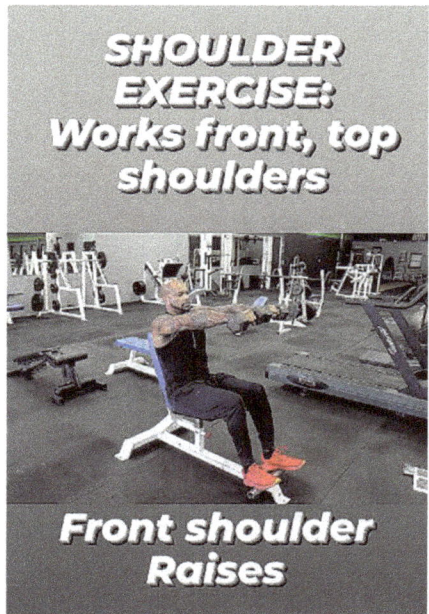

**SHOULDER EXERCISE:** Works front, top shoulders

**Front shoulder Raises**

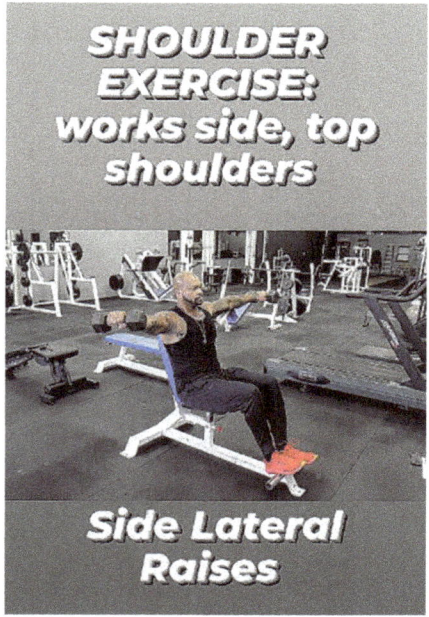

**SHOULDER EXERCISE:** works side, top shoulders

**Side Lateral Raises**

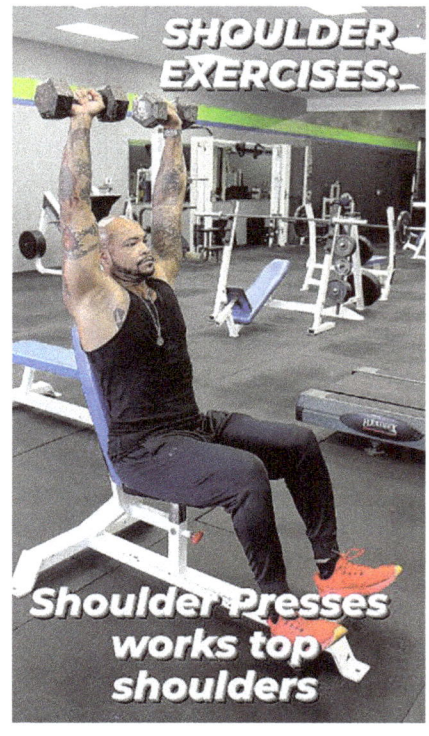

**SHOULDER EXERCISES:**

**Shoulder Presses works top shoulders**

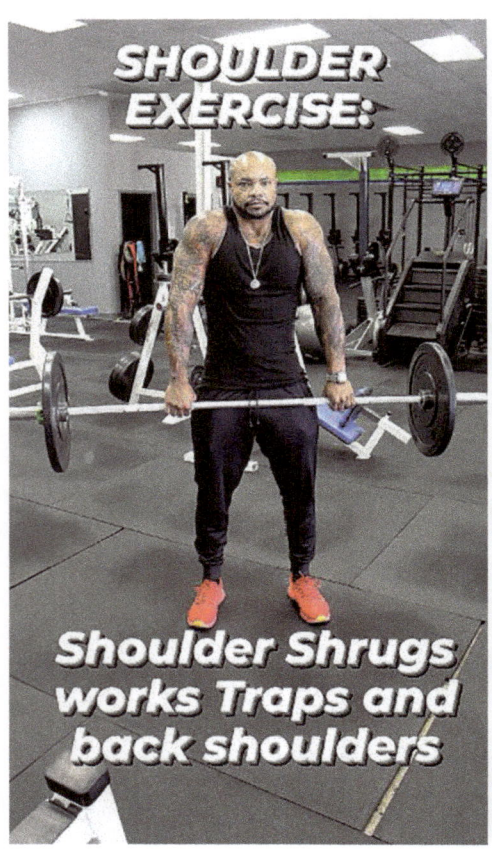

SHOULDER EXERCISE:

Shoulder Shrugs works Traps and back shoulders

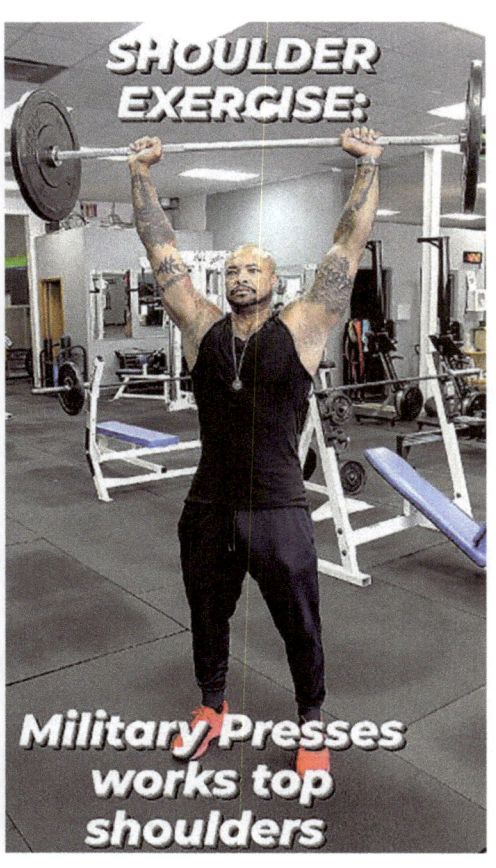

SHOULDER EXERCISE:

Military Presses works top shoulders

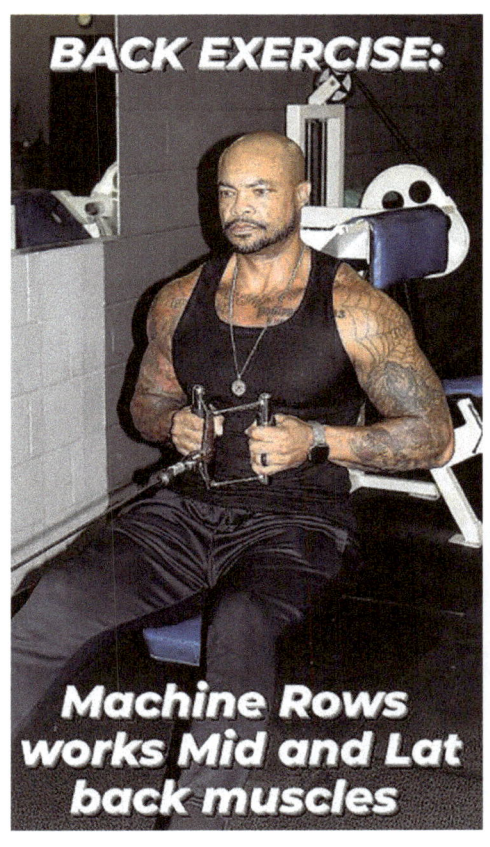

**BACK EXERCISE:**

**Machine Rows works Mid and Lat back muscles**

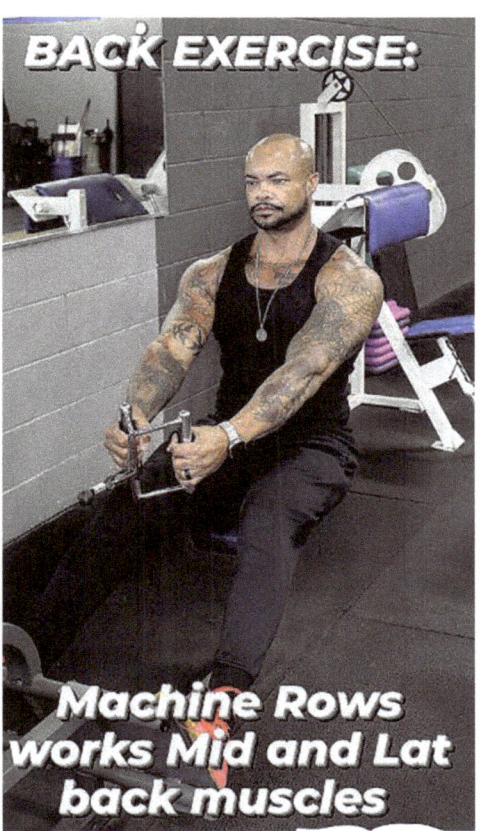

**BACK EXERCISE:**

**Machine Rows works Mid and Lat back muscles**

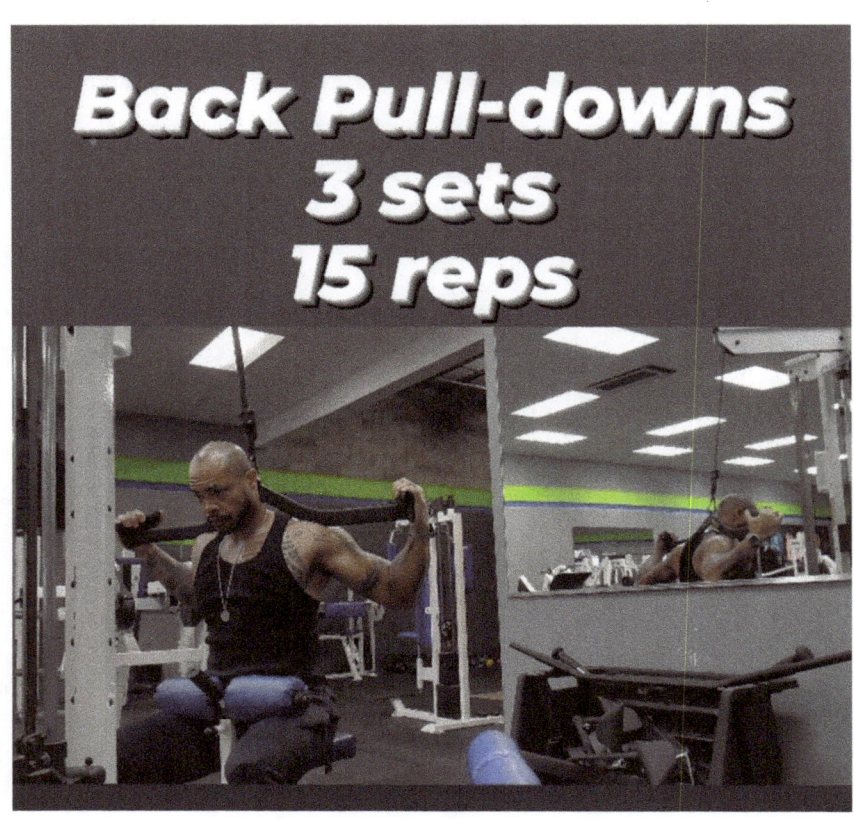

Back Pull-downs
3 sets
15 reps

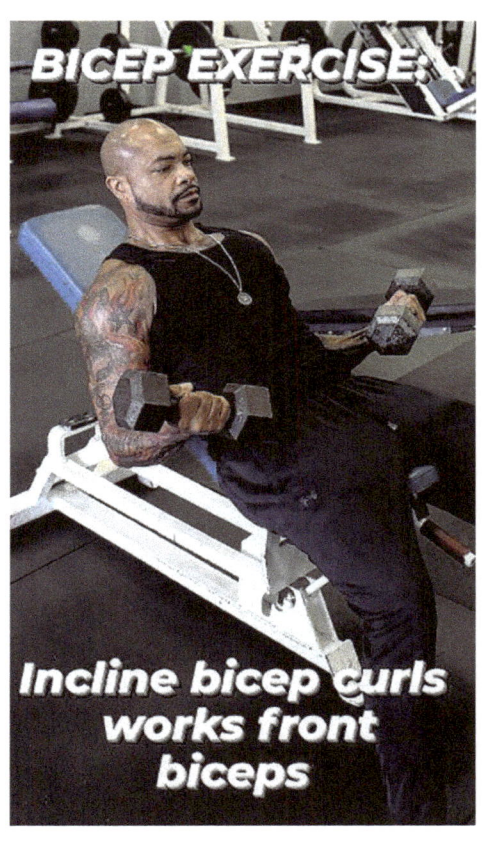

BICEP EXERCISE:

Incline bicep curls works front biceps

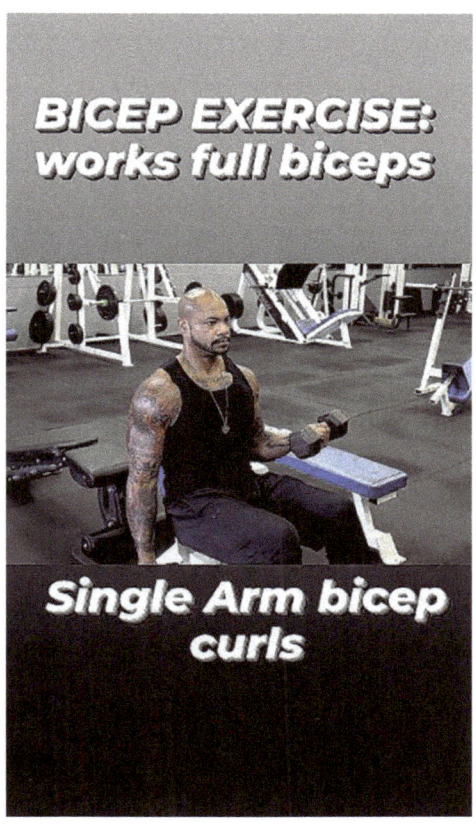

BICEP EXERCISE: works full biceps

Single Arm bicep curls

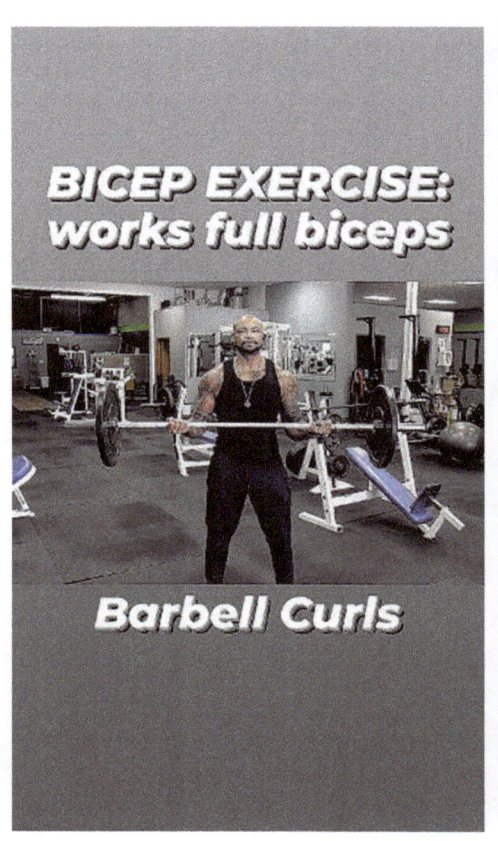

**BICEP EXERCISE:** *works full biceps*

**Barbell Curls**

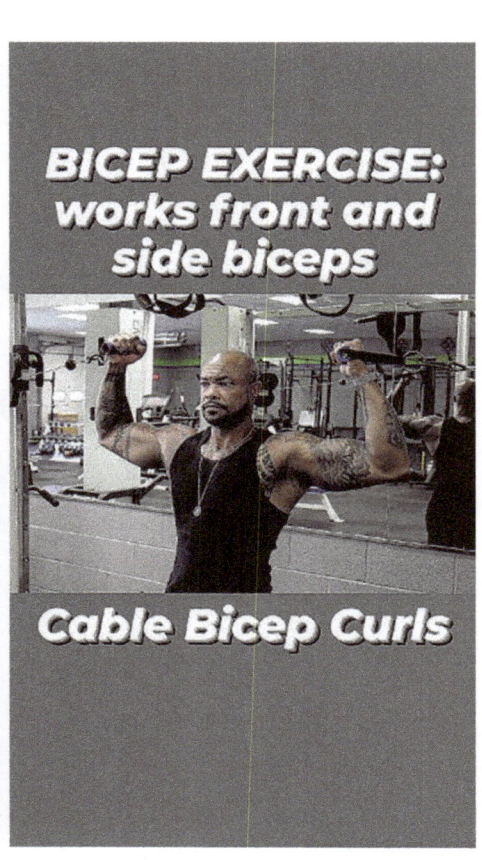

**BICEP EXERCISE:** *works front and side biceps*

**Cable Bicep Curls**

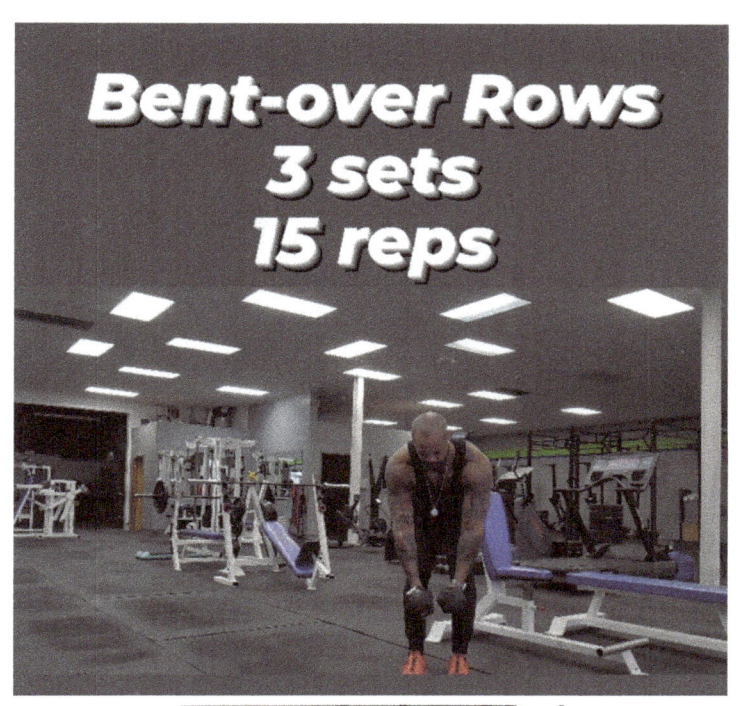

**Bent-over Rows**
**3 sets**
**15 reps**

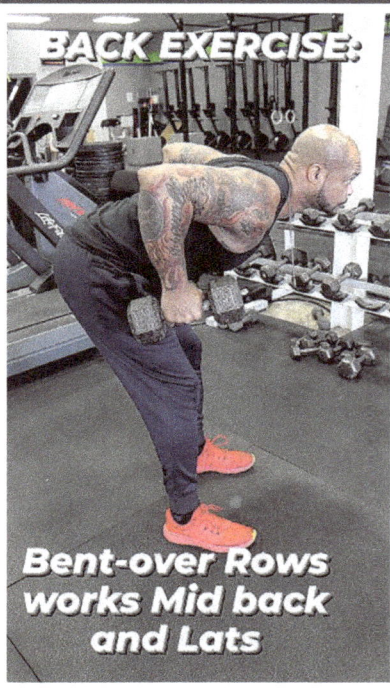

BACK EXERCISE:

**Bent-over Rows works Mid back and Lats**

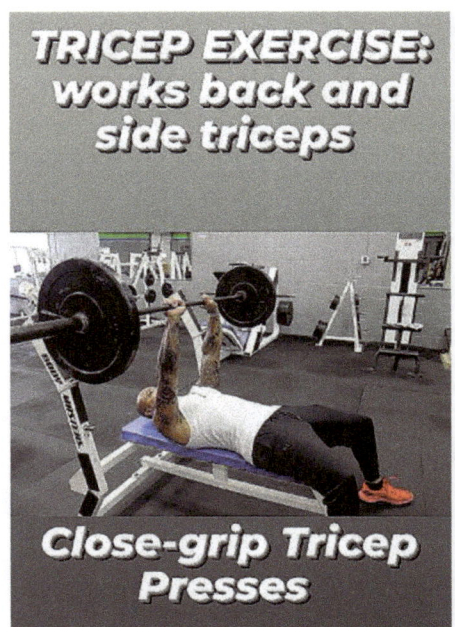

**TRICEP EXERCISE: works back and side triceps**

Close-grip Tricep Presses

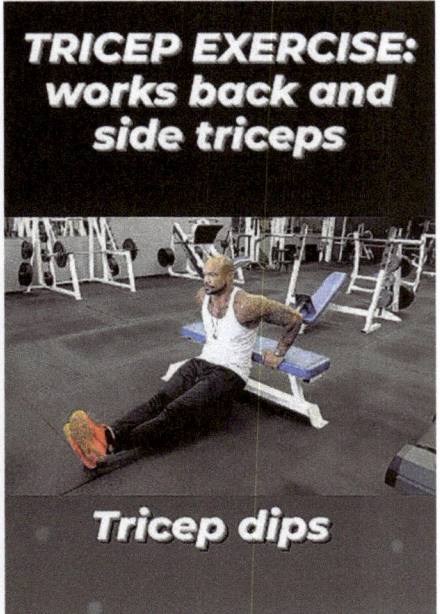

**TRICEP EXERCISE: works back and side triceps**

Tricep dips

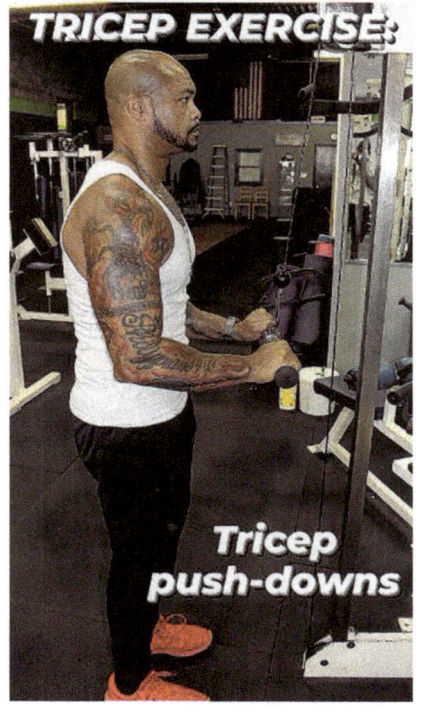

**TRICEP EXERCISE:**

Tricep push-downs

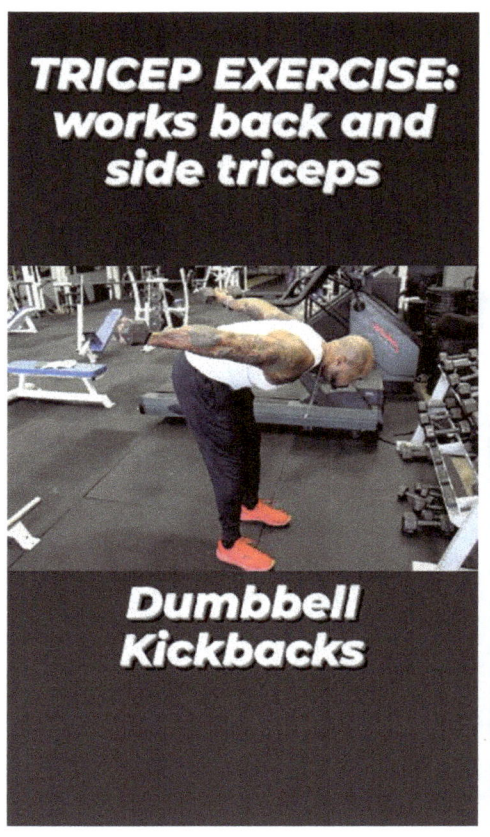

**TRICEP EXERCISE:** works back and side triceps

**Dumbbell Kickbacks**

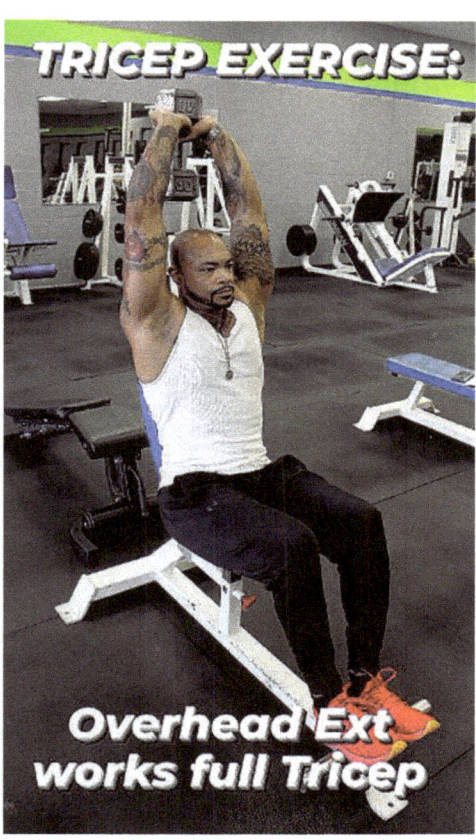

**TRICEP EXERCISE:**

**Overhead Ext works full Tricep**

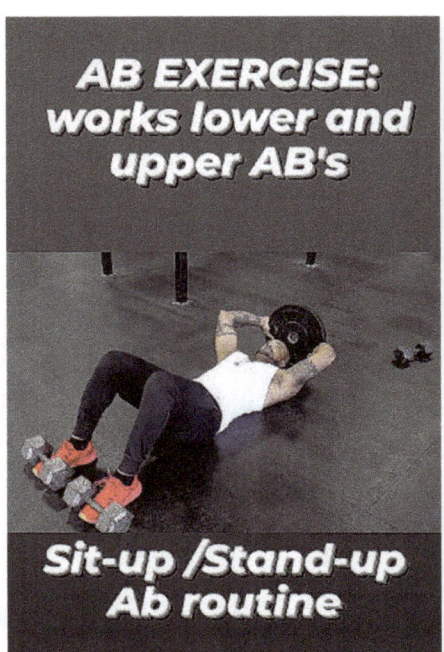

**AB EXERCISE:** works lower and upper AB's

Sit-up /Stand-up Ab routine

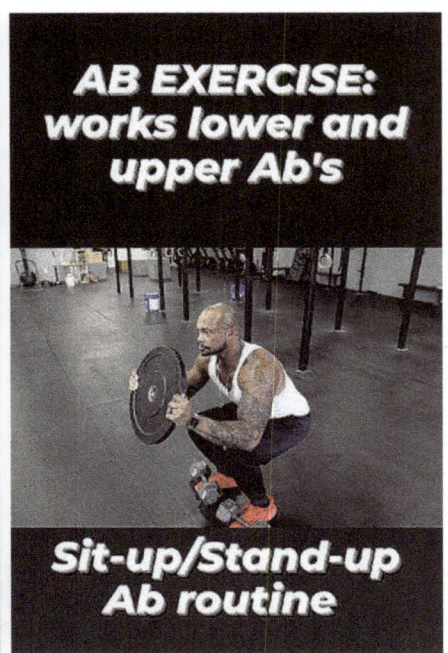

**AB EXERCISE:** works lower and upper Ab's

Sit-up/Stand-up Ab routine

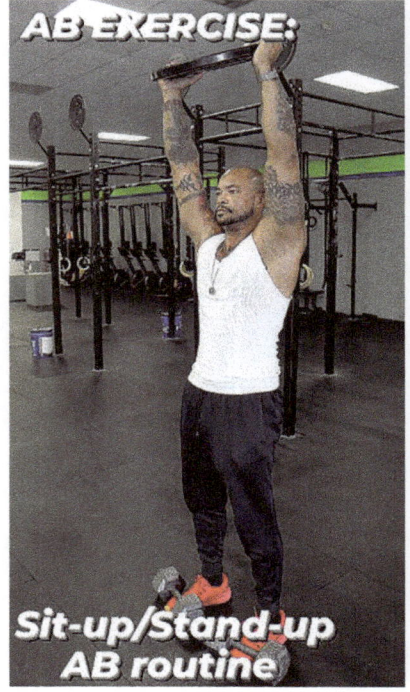

**AB EXERCISE:**

Sit-up/Stand-up AB routine

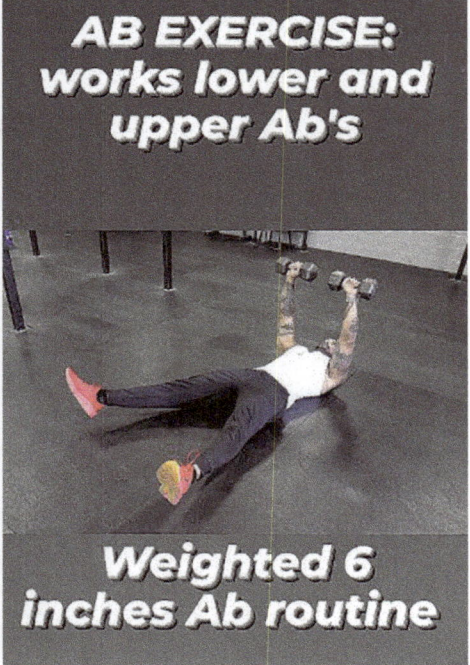

**AB EXERCISE:** works lower and upper Ab's

Weighted 6 inches Ab routine

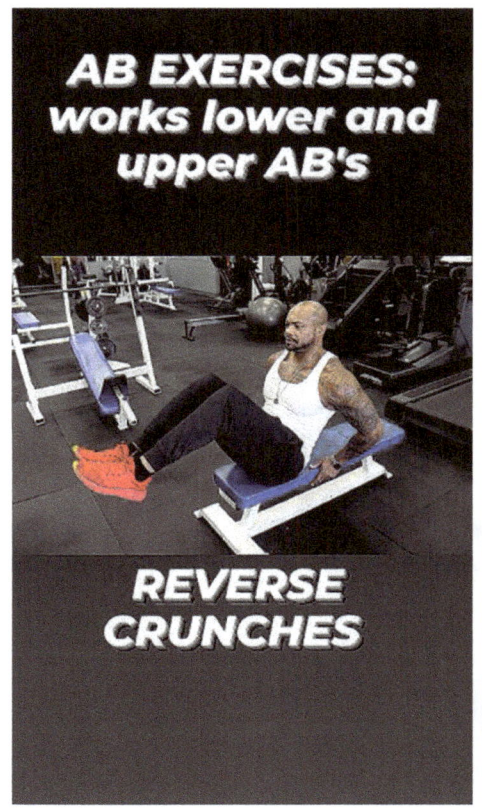

**AB EXERCISES: works lower and upper AB's**

**REVERSE CRUNCHES**

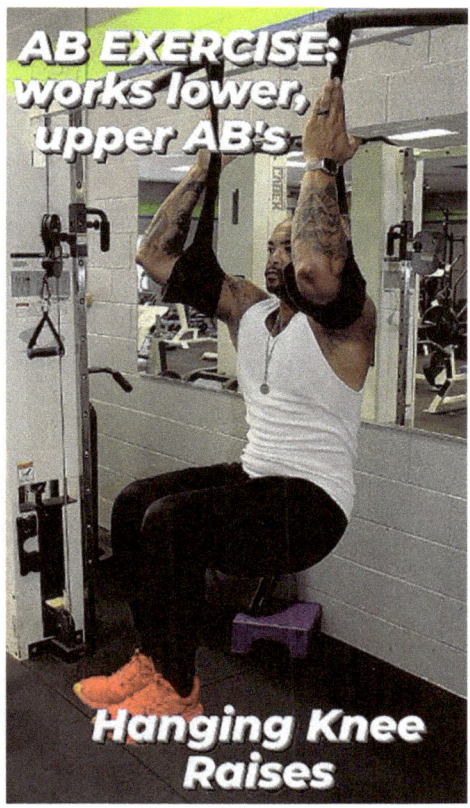

**AB EXERCISE: works lower, upper AB's**

**Hanging Knee Raises**

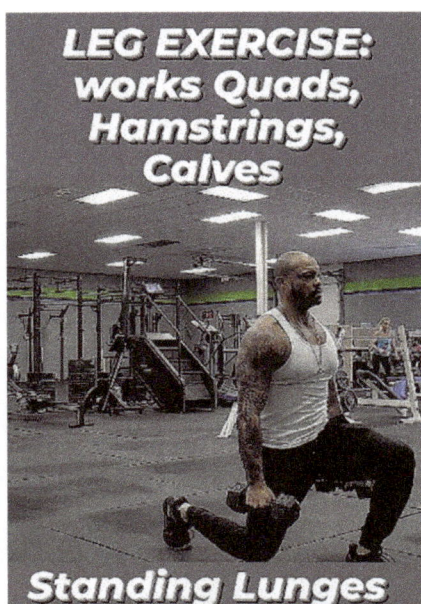

**LEG EXERCISE: works Quads, Hamstrings, Calves**

**Standing Lunges**

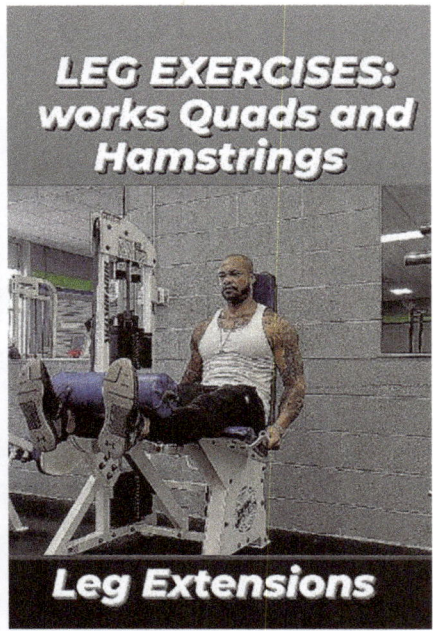

**LEG EXERCISES: works Quads and Hamstrings**

**Leg Extensions**

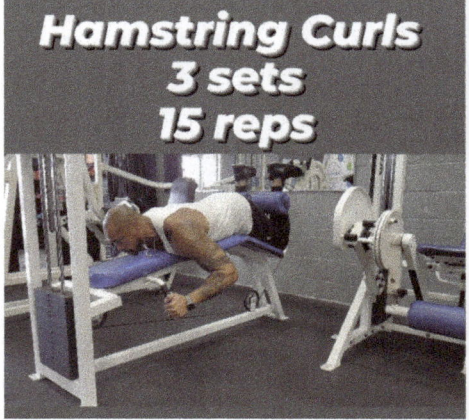

**Hamstring Curls 3 sets 15 reps**

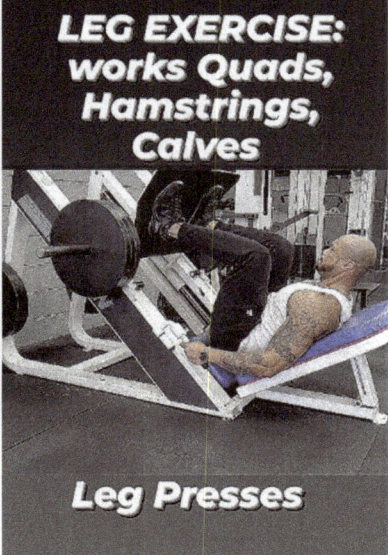

**LEG EXERCISE: works Quads, Hamstrings, Calves**

**Leg Presses**

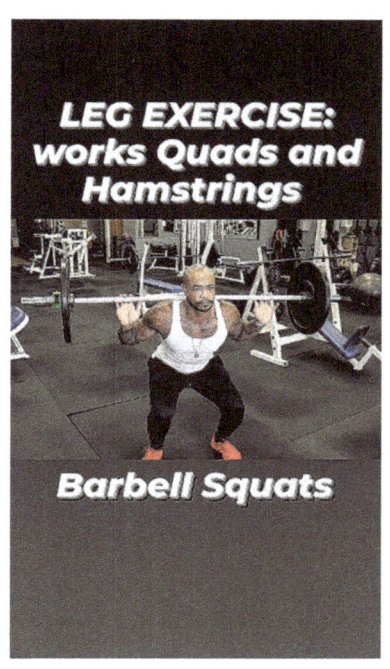

**LEG EXERCISE: works Quads and Hamstrings**

**Barbell Squats**

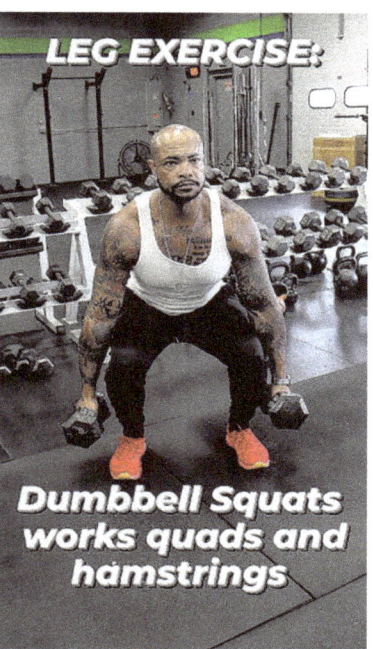

**LEG EXERCISE:**

**Dumbbell Squats works quads and hamstrings**

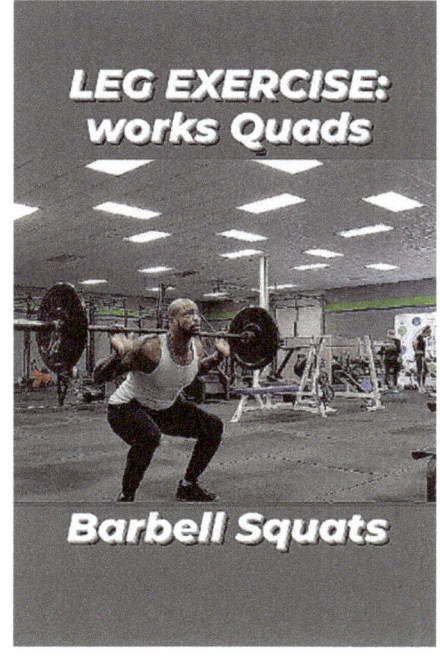

**LEG EXERCISE: works Quads**

**Barbell Squats**

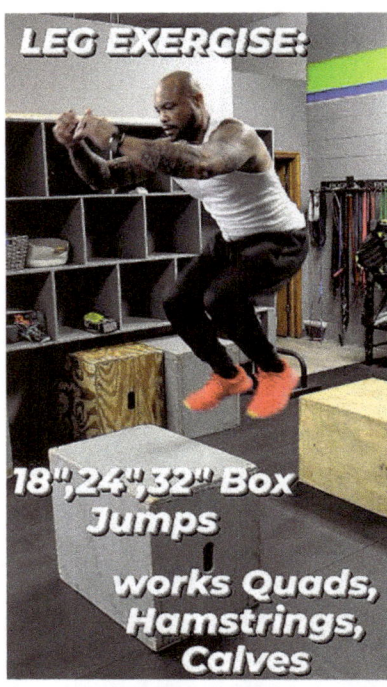

**LEG EXERCISE:**

18",24",32" Box Jumps

works Quads, Hamstrings, Calves

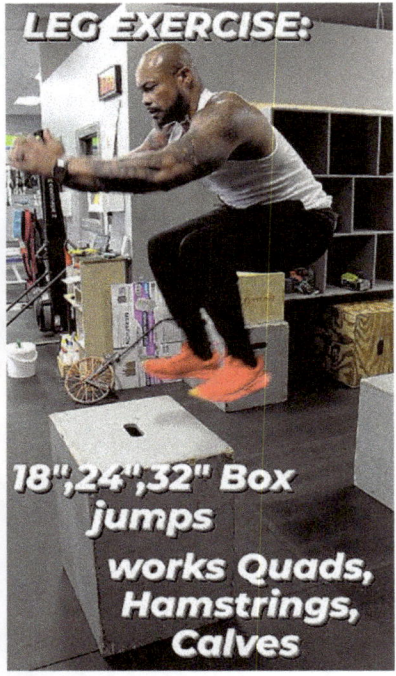

**LEG EXERCISE:**

18",24",32" Box jumps

works Quads, Hamstrings, Calves

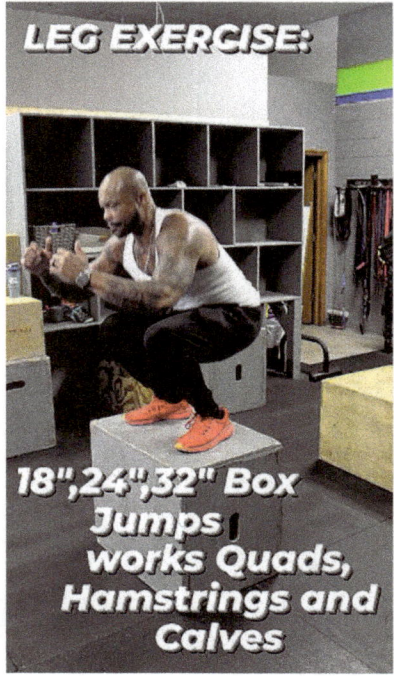

**LEG EXERCISE:**

18",24",32" Box Jumps works Quads, Hamstrings and Calves

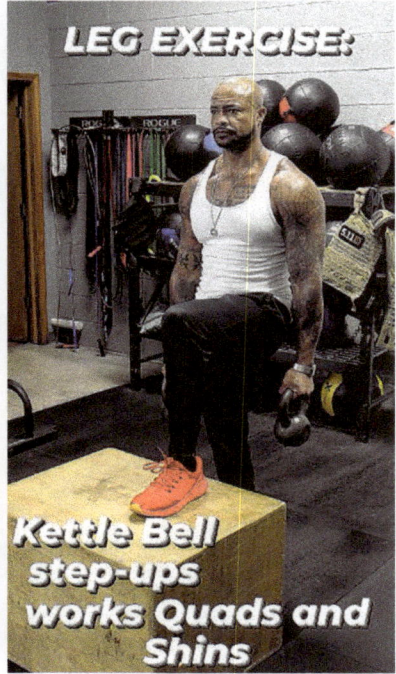

**LEG EXERCISE:**

Kettle Bell step-ups works Quads and Shins

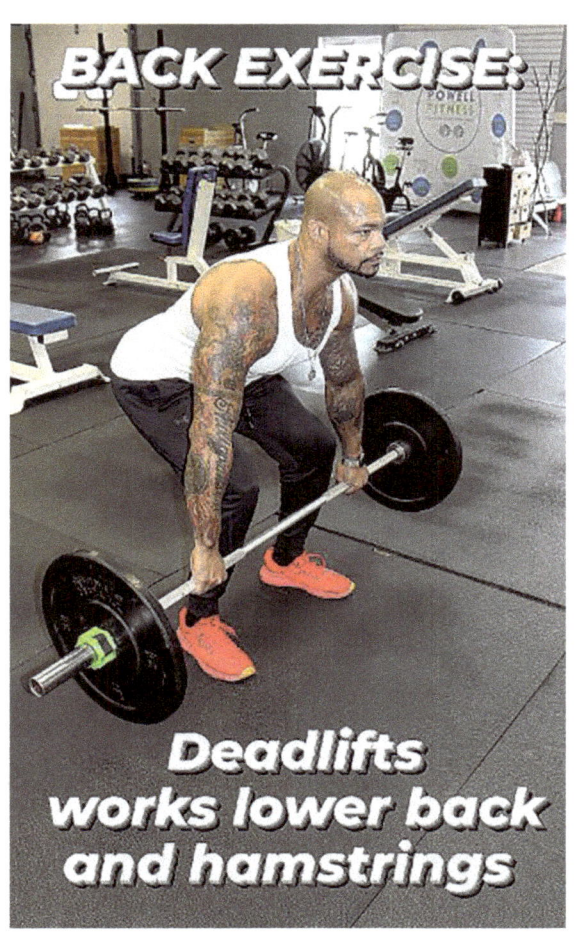

**BACK EXERCISE:**

**Deadlifts works lower back and hamstrings**

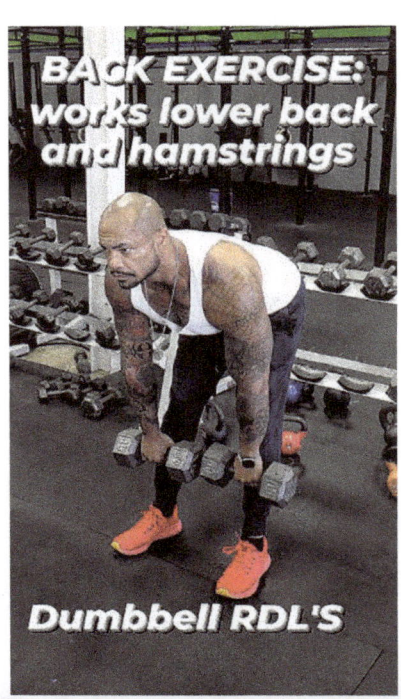

BACK EXERCISE: works lower back and hamstrings

Dumbbell RDL'S

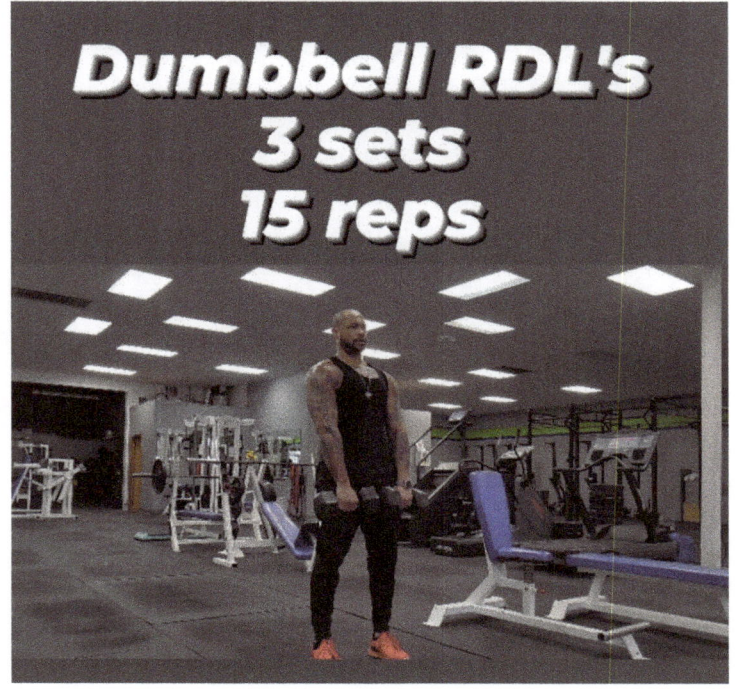

Dumbbell RDL's
3 sets
15 reps

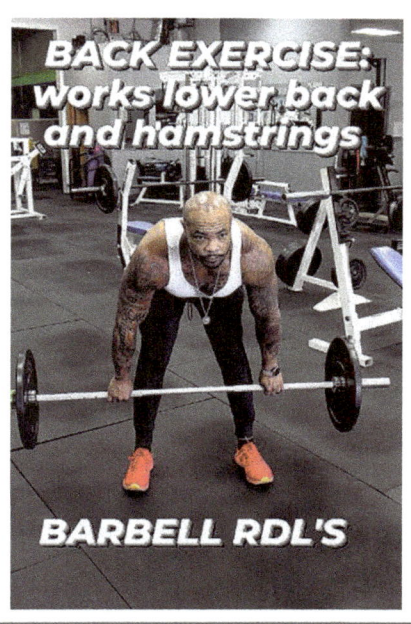

BARBELL RDL'S

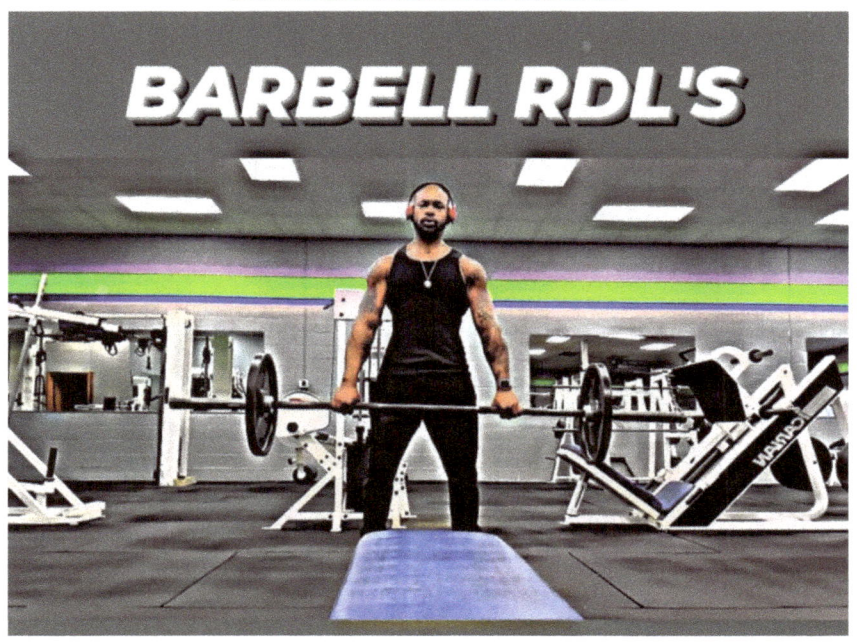

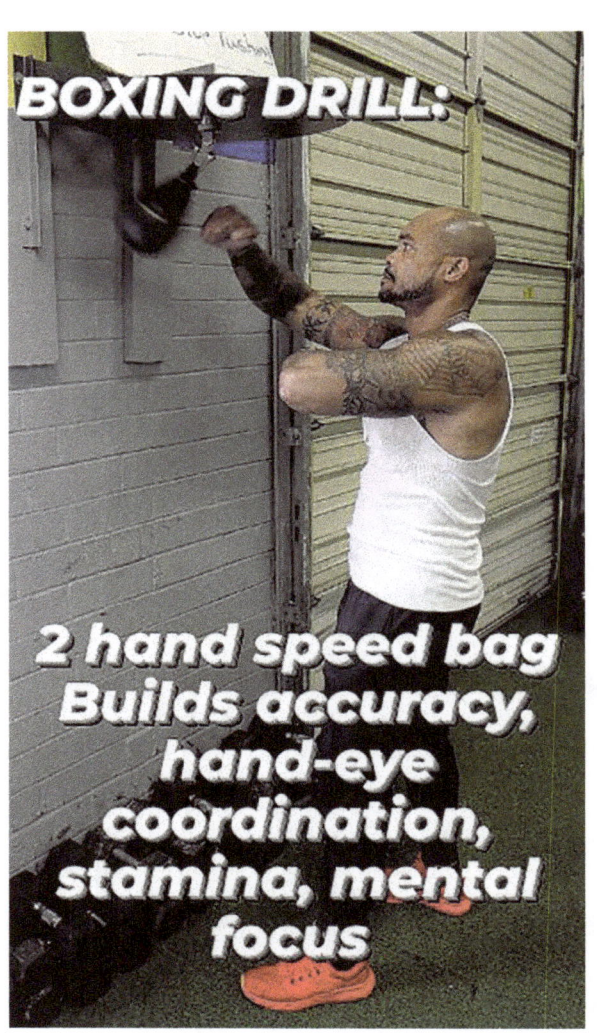

**BOXING DRILL:**

**2 hand speed bag Builds accuracy, hand-eye coordination, stamina, mental focus**

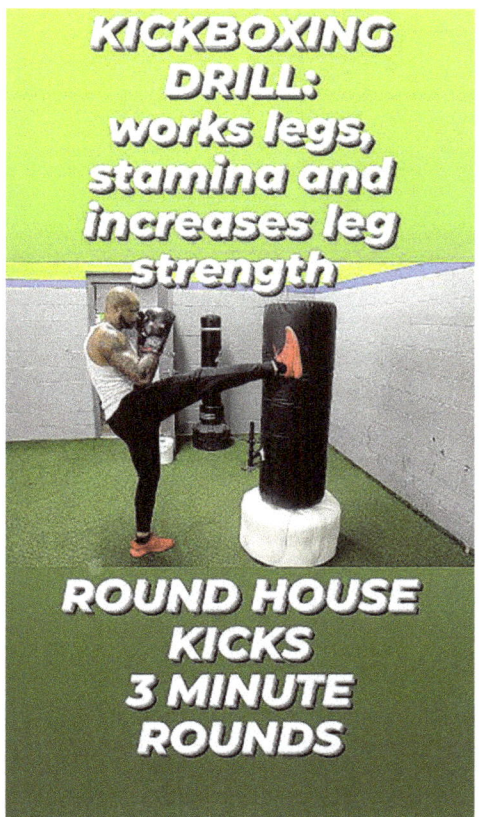

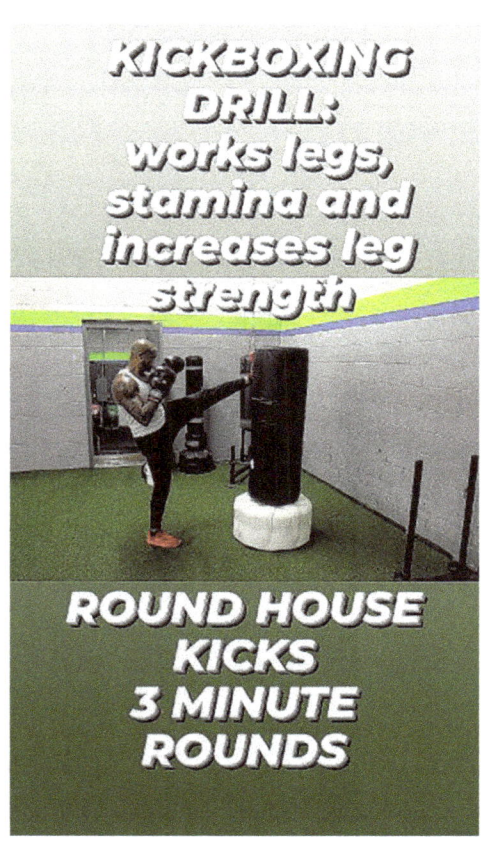

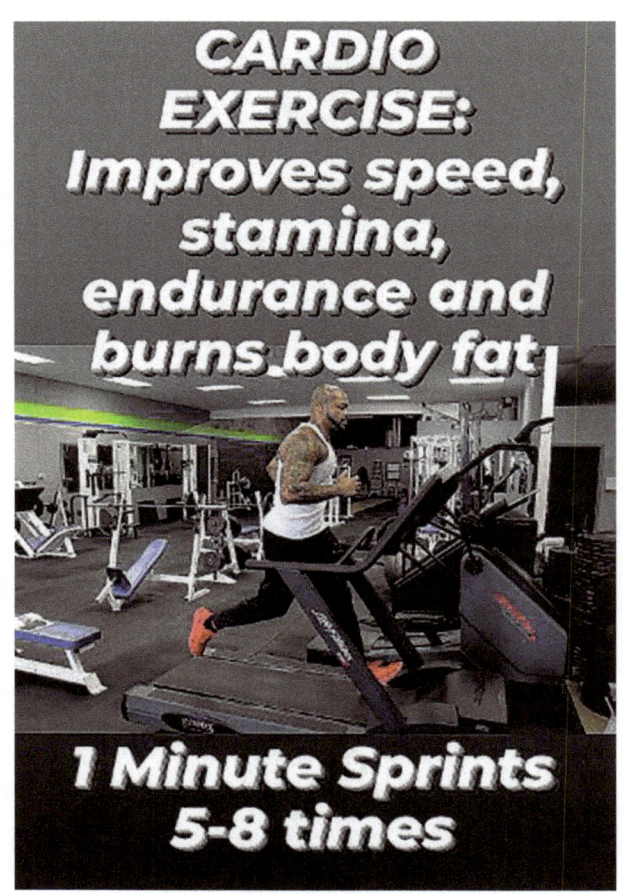

My experience with Mr. Webb has been phenomenal. I started working out in March 2020, and I have seen so much progress in my body, targeting areas and hitting my ideal weight goal. Mr. Webb is an excellent trainer, professional in helping you accomplish how to lose body fat, build muscle, and get toned without looking muscular. I encourage males and females to stick with desiring to be fit, healthy, and consistent. Always be cautious of how and what you eat. Abs are made in the kitchen and not the gym. You can do it. Mr. Webb is awesome. I highly recommend him for whatever goal you have pertaining to your health.

—Ms. Covington

I began training with Marcus Webb after completing cancer treatment and contracting COVID-19. I was quite weak. I am a sixty-plus older female, and Marcus understands and respects my limitations while challenging me to be my best. Initially, my goal was to gain enough strength to stand up from the floor without pulling myself up with the use of a chair. I exceeded my initial goal, and Marcus motivated me to become stronger with each training session while always placing emphasis on safety. Marcus is very reliable, which is important as I often train during my lunch hour. Despite his muscular and intimidating appearance, he is a kind and gentle man. I look forward to continuing my fitness journey with Marcus.

—Barbara M.

As a family doctor, I see different levels of fitness. My patients who work consistently at staying active are the ones who are healthy and happy. In my seventy-five years, I have tried all sorts of things and found that loss of motivation and injury have been my greatest barriers. I have worked with Marcus for years and can honestly say I feel better than I ever have. Marcus really knows his stuff, and his book will be an invaluable resource.

–Robert Thacker, MD, FACP

I have been very fortunate to have Marcus Webb as my personal fitness trainer for the past twelve years. He has taught me so much about what constitutes healthy eating. Marcus introduced me to intermittent fasting, which has been a game changer in my quest to stay healthy and avoid bad eating habits. Marcus is patient and understanding but encourages me to move out of my comfort zone and try a new workout technique, a heavier weight, or just one more rep. The result? I am stronger, trimmer, and healthier as a sixty-five-year-old woman than I was in my forties!

—Gail Williams, retired school teacher

I've been training with Marcus for three years, and at fifty-seven, I'm in the best shape I've been in since my twenties. He's created a training regimen that has combined both strength training and cardio and kept things fresh and motivating.

—Sam Larose

I've been training with Marcus for two years. He's motivational and knowledgeable and cares about his clients. He's gone above and beyond to help me reach my goals.

—Sandi Larose

Marcus inspires me to be the better version of myself. I've been working out with Marcus off and on for ten years now, and he has been very flexible with my work scheduling. Marcus creates a workout that is fun, energetic, and therapeutic; and he always mixes it up so I don't get bored. Although my favorite workout is boxing, Marcus incorporates weights and circuit training in my workouts to strengthen my body, which helps me be better in my boxing sessions! Marcus is the best.

—Savita Jailall, bank manager

Marcus is an incredible trainer, and I'm so grateful for his work. His encouragement and constant motivation pushed me to heights I never thought possible. He truly cares and goes above and beyond to help me achieve my fitness goals. He inspires me to be excellent!

—Martha Hundley

After my bone density scan showed signs of early osteopenia, my physician recommended I begin a weight-bearing exercise regimen. He was kind enough to recommend his personal trainer, Marcus, to me. I never exercised regularly and didn't quite [know] what to expect.

Marcus is incredibly knowledgeable in his field and very attentive, kind, and personable. He started me out with weight-bearing exercises and has gradually increased the weights as I grew stronger. Now I have much more strength and stamina throughout my days. I'm grateful to Marcus for all he does!

—Shari Massey

In 2007 Marcus came highly recommended via a friend who worked out with him, thus I decided to give him a try. When I began training with Marcus, my starting weight was 200 pounds. After training with Marcus, My weight dropped down to 173 pounds, which is the smallest I've ever been!

Marcus is an awesome trainer who makes [it] a point to listen to your physical and mental needs, concerns, and issues. He immediately recognizes your potential and continues to push you even when you think you don't have any more to give. Training with Marcus is easily one of the best decisions I've done for my overall health and well-being.

—Nasia Morris, essential hospital worker

I have been training with Marcus for years, and he has always been so positive and encouraging. His workouts are customized to each person based on their abilities. He also takes into consideration any limitations you may have and create a workout plan to fit your needs. Marcus also helps with your food plan and supports you in all aspects of your fitness and health journey. I have referred several people over the years and will continue to do so. He's definitely the best! I appreciate all he has done for me!

—Dawn Wood, dental hygienist

I have been training with Marcus for the past thirteen-plus years. My initial goal when I started to train with Marcus was to lose weight, which I did, and I looked the best I've ever had in my life. I was able to maintain a healthy lifestyle throughout those years while trying out other types of workouts such as boxing and cycling but always found myself training with Marcus. He's always providing new training styles that never get old or stale. He changes things up, making our workouts interesting and, most of all, challenging and effective. I aim to continue training with Marcus for years to come and would recommend him in a heartbeat.

—Telmawatee "Sabrina" Jailall, business owner (Selena's Fine Lingerie Boutique)

# About the Author

My name is Marcus Webb. I've been in the fitness industry for over thirty years. I took my first weight-lifting class at the YMCA at age ten and fell in love with working out ever since. I was influenced by my father as well. He lifted weights a lot and played basketball, so I wanted to follow in his footsteps. I played basketball and various sports and lifted weights at an early age up to now. I got first place in my first bodybuilding show in 1999, and that I also have trained competitive men and women bodybuilders for bodybuilding shows. Fitness has really changed my life for the better. I am truly grateful. I am from Roanoke, Virginia, but now reside in Greensboro, North Carolina, as a fitness trainer.

I am a certified fitness trainer and boxing coach. I have coached a wide variety of individuals from housewives, kids, general workers, police officers, firefighters, doctors, attorneys, military staffers to pro athletes. I can create an effective fitness program for anyone. I have a fitness certification through *International Fitness Association* and a boxing coach certification through the legendary Tony Spain, a former Golden Glove champion.

Fitness is my life until I die! It's deeply instilled in me since I was a kid. I live and breathe it every day! I am truly grateful for fitness. Now let's *get that work*!